BATTLING COVID-19

Invisible INVASION

The COVID-19 Pandemic Begins

MARIE BENDER

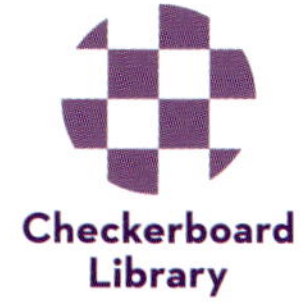

Checkerboard Library

An Imprint of Abdo Publishing
abdobooks.com

abdobooks.com

Printed in the United States of America, North Mankato, Minnesota
102020
012021

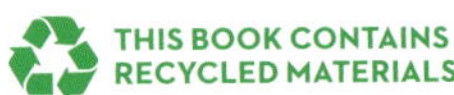

Design: Sarah DeYoung, Mighty Media, Inc.
Production: Mighty Media, Inc.
Editor: Jessica Rusick
Cover Photograph: Shutterstock Images
Interior Photographs: ANTHONY BEHAR/SIPA USA/AP Images, p. 23; Jens B'ttner/AP Images, p. 21; Shutterstock Images, pp. 5, 6, 7, 9, 10, 11, 13, 17, 19, 27, 29; South_agency/iStockphoto, pp. 6 (bottom), 25
Design Elements: Shutterstock Images

Library of Congress Control Number: 2020940286

Publisher's Cataloging-in-Publication Data
Names: Bender, Marie, author.
Title: Invisible invasion: the COVID-19 pandemic begins / by Marie Bender
Other title: the COVID-19 pandemic begins
Description: Minneapolis, Minnesota : Abdo Publishing, 2021 | Series: Battling COVID-19 | Includes online resources and index
Identifiers: ISBN 9781532194290 (lib. bdg.) | ISBN 9781098213657 (ebook)
Subjects: LCSH: COVID-19 (Disease)--Juvenile literature. | Communicable diseases--Prevention--Juvenile literature. | Distance education--Juvenile literature. | Social distance--Juvenile literature. | Hygiene--Juvenile literature.
Classification: DDC 614.44--dc23

Contents

COVID-19 Invasion

On December 31, 2019, the world started hearing about a mysterious disease in Wuhan, China. Dozens of people were falling ill. But, no one knew why. Doctors and scientists in China worked to discover the cause. In early January 2020, they announced that the disease was caused by a new coronavirus. The disease became known as COVID-19.

On January 23, Chinese officials imposed a **lockdown** in Wuhan. They closed businesses, schools, and public transportation. Officials hoped this would keep the disease from spreading. But it was too late. People who had already left Wuhan brought COVID-19 to other areas of China. From there, the disease spread to other countries.

By late January, nearly 10,000 people had been **infected** with the coronavirus. And, 213 people had died. By the first week of March, about 90,000 people had the disease. Deaths had risen to 3,000. On March 11, 2020, the **World Health Organization (WHO)** declared COVID-19 a **pandemic**. The COVID-19 invasion was well underway.

WHAT IS A CORONAVIRUS?

Coronaviruses are a large group of viruses that cause **respiratory** illnesses. Most coronaviruses exist only in animals. However, several have spread from animals to humans. The coronavirus discovered in Wuhan is called severe acute respiratory syndrome coronavirus 2 (SARS-CoV-2). It causes a disease called coronavirus disease 2019, or COVID-19. COVID-19 spreads when saliva droplets pass from person to person. This can happen when someone coughs, sneezes, sings, breathes, or talks. Most people with COVID-19 do not suffer serious **symptoms**. But some people develop life-threatening problems. Because of this, the virus is viewed as a threat to world health.

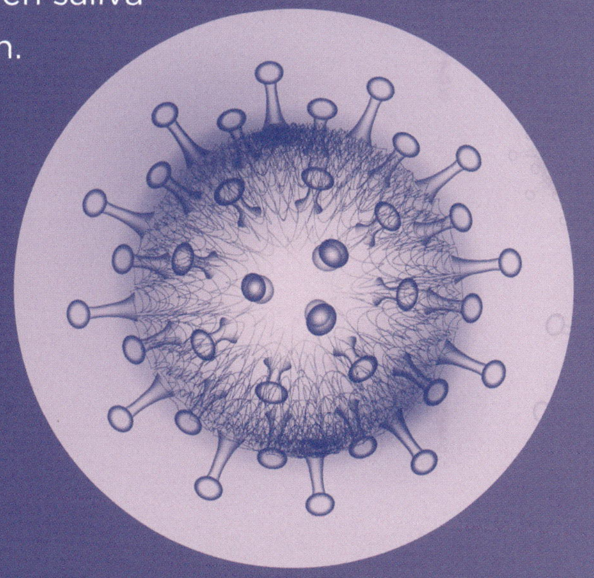

TIMELINE

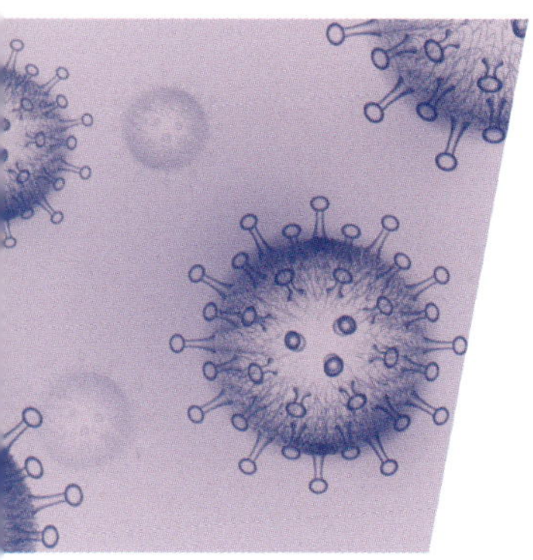

DECEMBER 31, 2019

Cases of a mysterious new disease are reported in Wuhan, China. The disease, COVID-19, is caused by a new virus called SARS-CoV-2.

JANUARY 21, 2020

The first COVID-19 case is reported in the United States.

JANUARY 23, 2020

Chinese officials close the city of Wuhan to stop COVID-19 from spreading.

JANUARY 31, 2020

US President Donald Trump declares COVID-19 a public health emergency.

EARLY MARCH 2020

The United States reaches 500 COVID-19 cases. Worldwide, 90,000 people have been infected with COVID-19 and 3,000 have died.

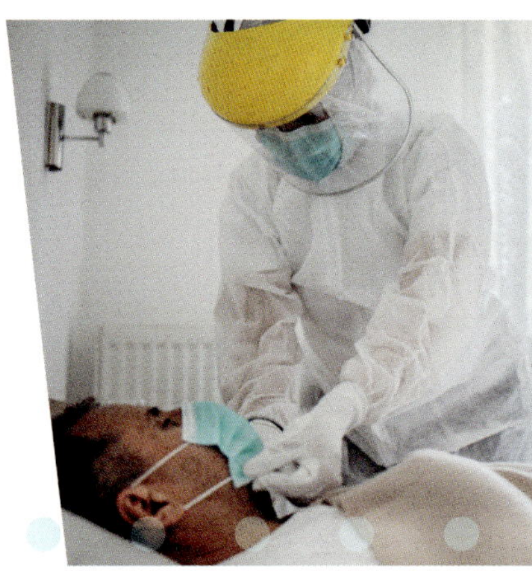

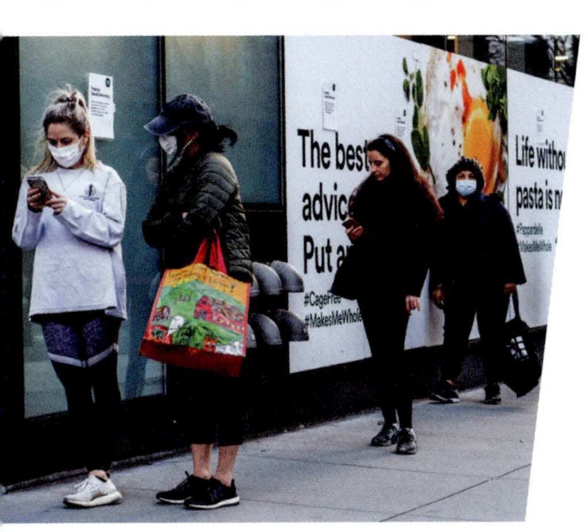

MARCH 11, 2020

The World Health Organization (WHO) declares COVID-19 a pandemic.

MARCH 13, 2020

President Trump declares COVID-19 a national emergency.

MARCH 15, 2020

The Centers for Disease Control and Prevention (CDC) encourages social distancing and recommends limiting gatherings of 50 or more people.

LATE APRIL 2020

COVID-19 cases have been reported in most countries around the world.

EARLY JUNE 2020

There are nearly 6.4 million confirmed COVID-19 cases worldwide. The disease has killed more than 380,000 people.

OCTOBER 2020

There are 33 million COVID-19 cases worldwide. One million people have died from the disease.

Worldwide Infection

The first COVID-19 cases outside China were in nearby countries. Between January 13 and January 20, Thailand, Japan, and South Korea reported four total COVID-19 cases.

Italy was one of the first European countries to have a COVID-19 **outbreak**. By February 23, the country had more than 150 cases. Officials closed schools and canceled public events. Travel between towns was **restricted**. Other European countries also imposed stern travel and border controls.

Despite these efforts, COVID-19 continued to spread. By March, the disease had taken over countries on the other side of the world, including the United States.

COVID-19 AND RACISM

Some Asians and people of Asian descent experienced racism during the COVID-19 **pandemic**. This is because the virus **originated** in China. In the United States and other countries, Asian people were the victims of hate crimes. They were harassed, attacked, and blamed for spreading the virus.

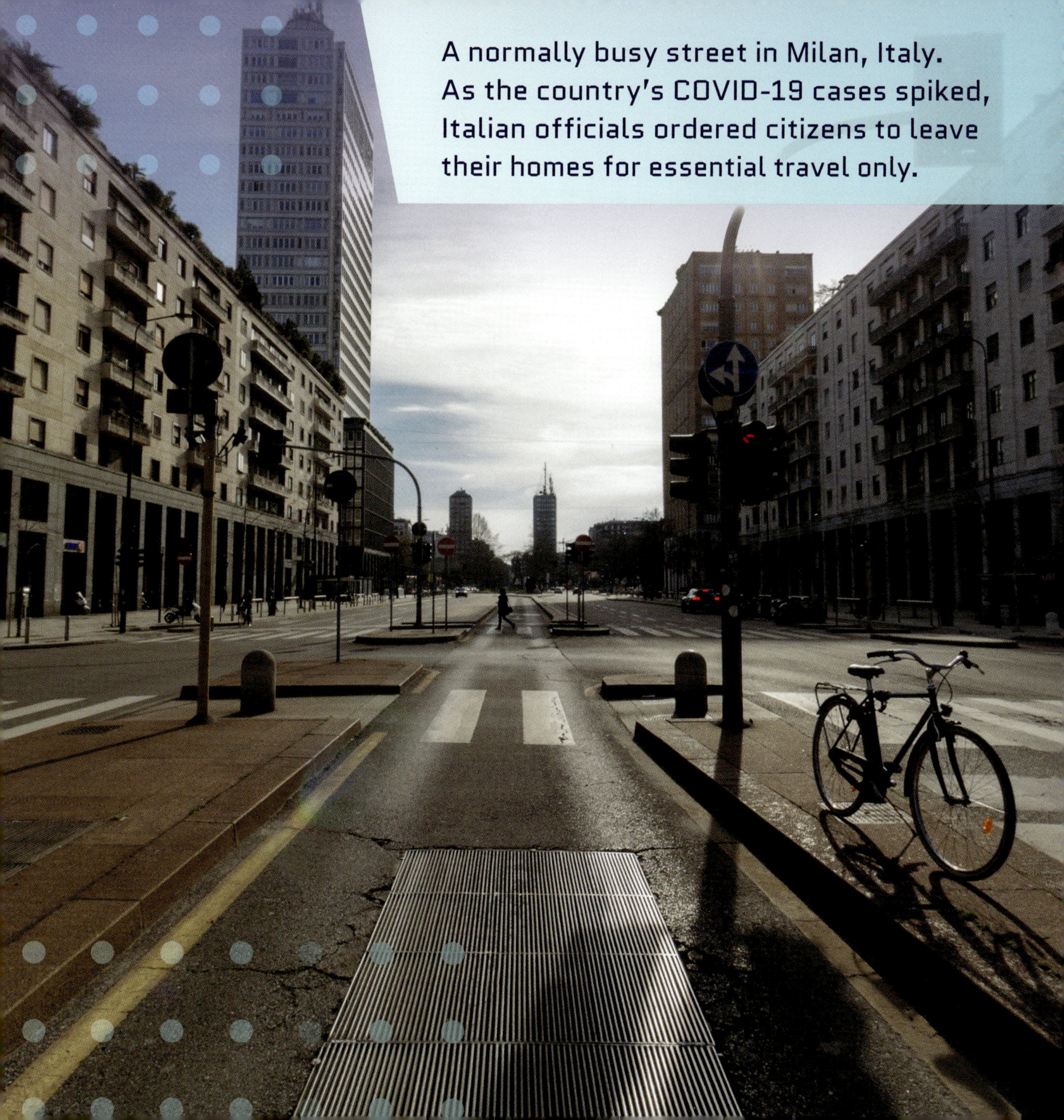

A normally busy street in Milan, Italy. As the country's COVID-19 cases spiked, Italian officials ordered citizens to leave their homes for essential travel only.

Global Impact

SWEDEN

Sweden's first COVID-19 case was confirmed on February 4. Officials asked citizens to work from home if possible. They also limited gatherings of more than 50 people. However, unlike most other countries, Sweden did not impose a **lockdown.** Schools and restaurants remained open.

UNITED KINGDOM

The first case of COVID-19 in the United Kingdom was confirmed on January 31. The country went into lockdown on March 23. This was much later than other countries. Under the lockdown, public gatherings of more than two people were prohibited.

SOUTH KOREA

COVID-19 first spread to South Korea on January 20. But the country did not go into **lockdown.** Instead, South Korea focused on testing its citizens for the virus. A smartphone app allowed **infected** people to report where they had traveled recently. This helped officials trace the spread of the virus. It also helped warn others of potential exposure.

SOUTH AFRICA

South Africa's first case of COVID-19 was reported on March 5. The country soon imposed a lockdown. At the time, it was one of the most severe lockdowns in the world. Most travel was **restricted.** And, everyone was required to wear masks in public.

Invading the United States

The first case of COVID-19 in the United States had been reported on January 21. It was in Washington State. The **infected** man had just traveled from Wuhan. Within ten days, there were several other cases in the United States.

On January 31, US President Donald Trump declared COVID-19 a public health emergency. He also announced that most travelers from China would not be allowed to enter the country. These **restrictions** were later expanded to include travelers from several other countries. The bans excluded US citizens and their immediate family members.

By early March, the United States had 500 cases. Most were in Washington, California, and New York. On March 13, Trump declared COVID-19 a national emergency. This allowed the government to use emergency funds to help fight the virus.

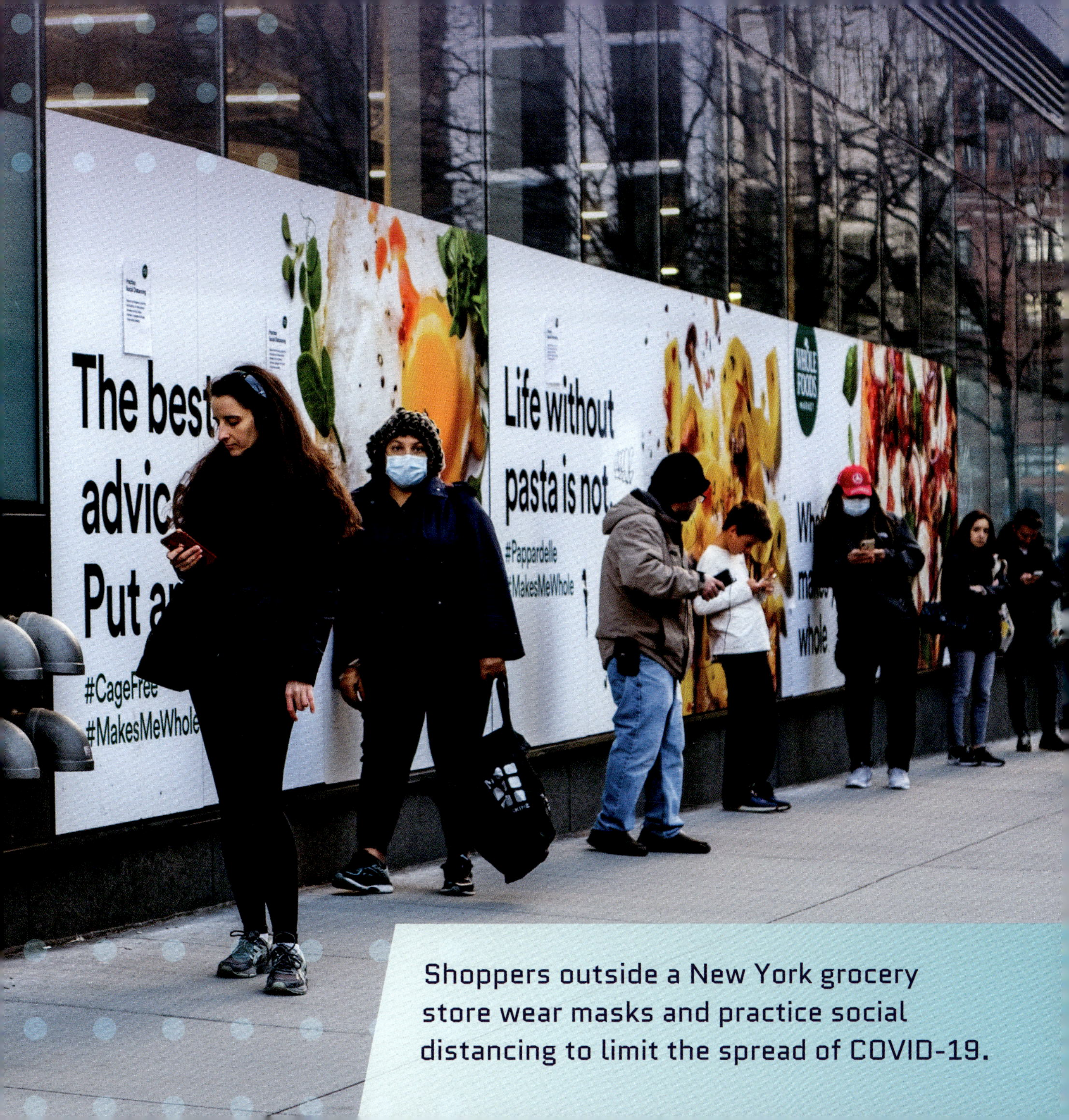

Shoppers outside a New York grocery store wear masks and practice social distancing to limit the spread of COVID-19.

On March 15, the **Centers for Disease Control and Prevention (CDC)** recommended that gatherings be kept to fewer than 50 people. The CDC also encouraged people to practice social distancing. This meant staying at least six feet (2 m) away from others.

Meanwhile, US governors and other local leaders were responding to the **crisis**. They issued orders for residents to stay at home, or shelter in place. California, Illinois, and New York were

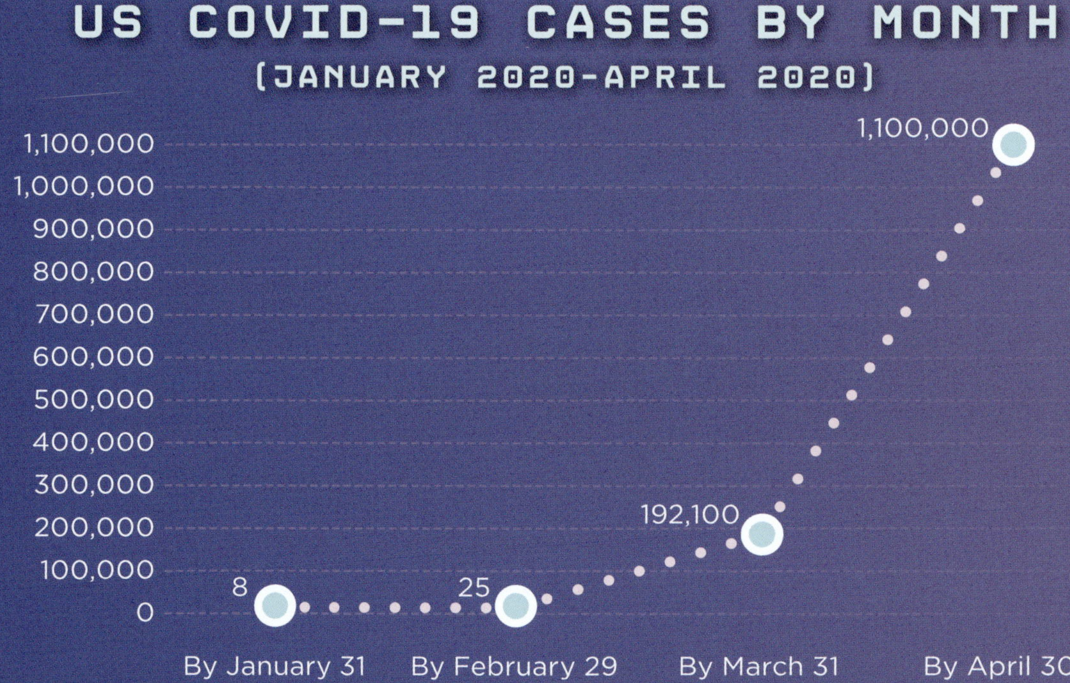

the first states to have such policies. By the first week of April, most other states had followed suit.

Many businesses had to close under the stay-at-home orders. Others could only offer delivery and pick-up services. Businesses that were considered **essential** could stay open. These included grocery stores, gas stations, and hospitals.

People who could do their jobs from home were able to continue working. Unfortunately, this wasn't possible for many people. So, millions of people lost their jobs. Schools across the country also closed. Students and teachers did their best to continue lessons online. But, graduation ceremonies and other school events had to be canceled.

Living under these new conditions wasn't easy. Some people grew bored or lonely. And many who lost their jobs faced financial trouble. However, many people felt that the sacrifices were necessary to stop the spread of COVID-19.

Source and Spread

By late April 2020, most countries had reported COVID-19 cases. Wuhan was the location of the first **infection**. But there was debate about the actual source of the virus. Scientists determined that SARS-CoV-2 **originated** in bats. However, coronaviruses aren't transferred directly from bats to people. So, scientists believe the new coronavirus was first transferred from a bat to another animal. The virus was then transferred to humans.

Many early COVID-19 cases were traced to a wet market in Wuhan. A wet market is a place where people sell fruits, vegetables, and live or recently slaughtered animals. At first, some scientists believed an animal at the wet market spread the SARS-CoV-2 virus to humans. However, new investigations showed the virus may not have originated from the wet market.

In the meantime, scientists learned exactly how the SARS-CoV-2 virus spread. When an infected person sneezes or coughs, tiny droplets containing the virus fly from their mouth or nose. Another person can become infected if they come into contact with the droplets.

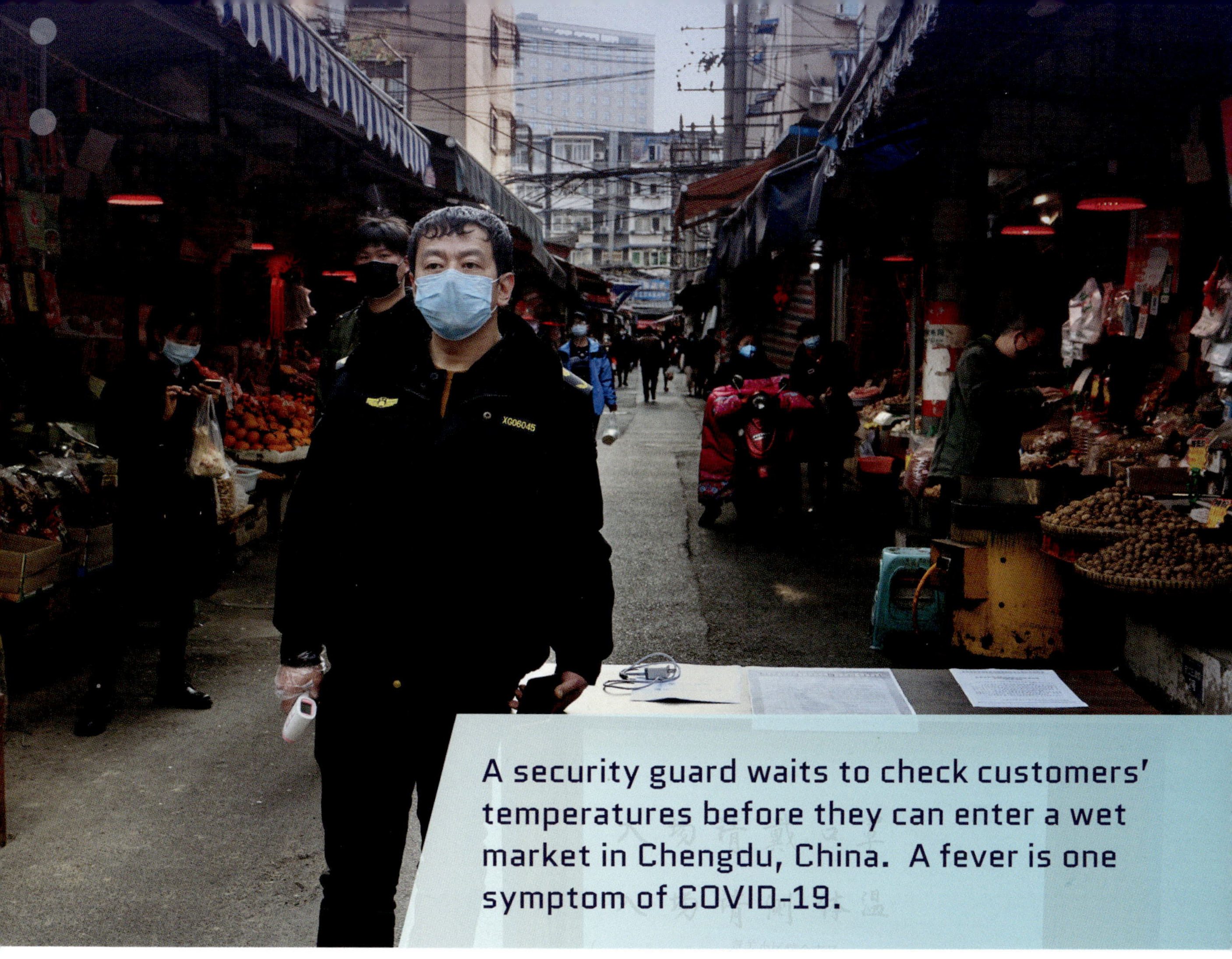

A security guard waits to check customers' temperatures before they can enter a wet market in Chengdu, China. A fever is one symptom of COVID-19.

Transfer of the coronavirus from person to person is called community spread. There are several ways to slow community spread. These include social distancing, washing hands, and wearing masks.

Symptoms and Testing

Social distancing and stay-at-home orders helped slow the spread of COVID-19. However, people continued to get sick. Many were healthcare workers treating COVID-19 patients. Others were people who worked in stores, at meatpacking plants, or as mail carriers.

The main **symptoms** of COVID-19 are coughing and difficulty breathing. Other symptoms include fever, chills, aches, sore throat, and loss of taste or smell. Many people experienced a mild case of the disease. They recovered at home. Others experienced severe symptoms. They had to be cared for in hospitals.

A person could be tested for COVID-19 in two ways. These were viral tests and **antibody** tests. A viral test determined

STEM CONNECTION

Scientists believe some people **infected** by COVID-19 are asymptomatic. This means they do not show symptoms, but the virus is active in their bodies. Asymptomatic carriers can still infect others with COVID-19. Without widespread testing, it is difficult to determine how many people are asymptomatic.

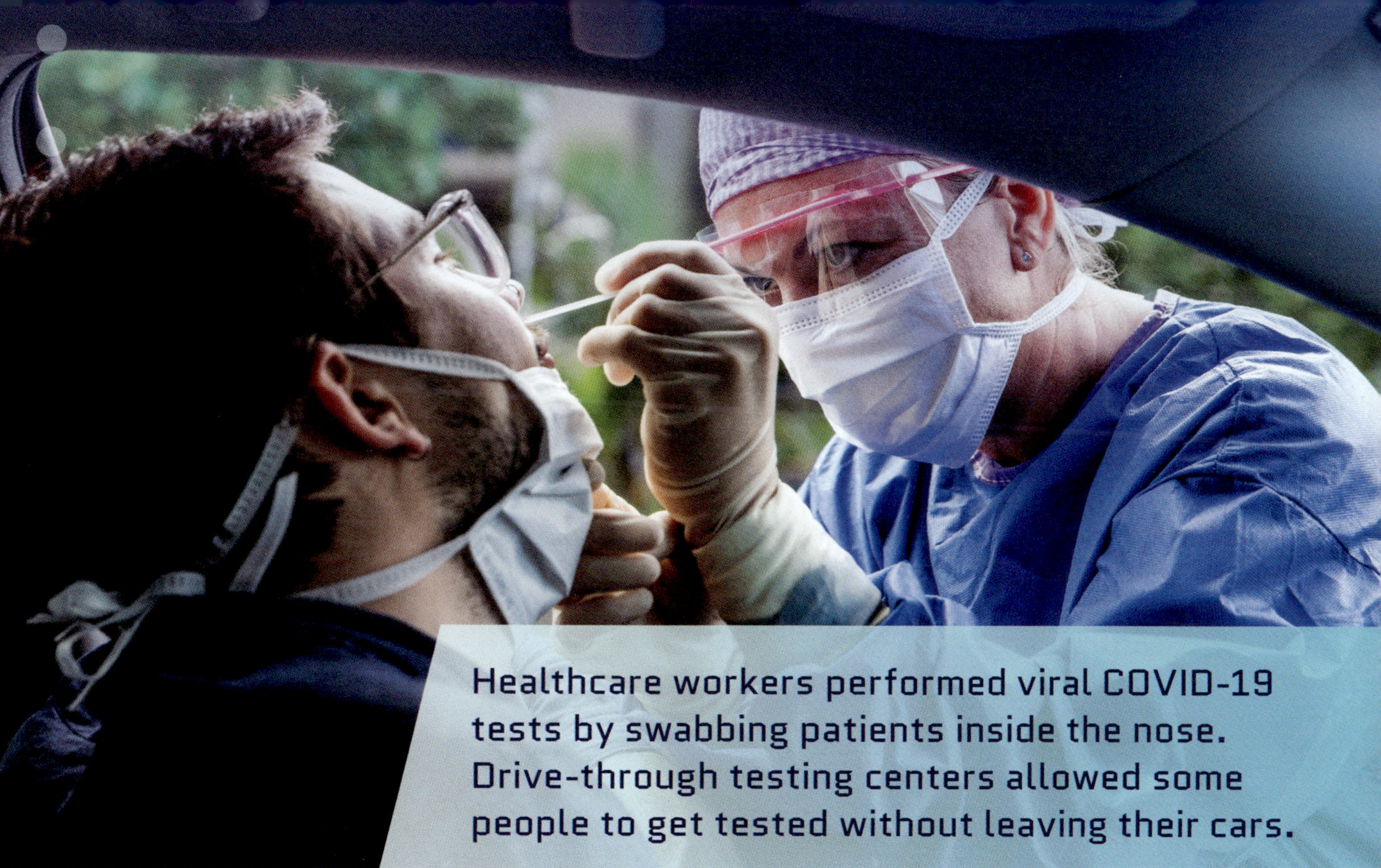

Healthcare workers performed viral COVID-19 tests by swabbing patients inside the nose. Drive-through testing centers allowed some people to get tested without leaving their cars.

whether someone was **infected** by the coronavirus. An **antibody** test determined whether someone had been infected but wasn't any longer.

Early in the **pandemic**, the United States faced widespread testing **shortages**. So, not everyone who experienced COVID-19 **symptoms** could get tested. Priority was given to healthcare workers. Tests were also given to those at high risk of developing a severe case of COVID-19.

Deadly Infection

Several factors can contribute to someone developing a serious case of COVID-19. People with existing medical conditions are at risk. These conditions include **asthma**, high blood pressure, and liver disease. People over 65 years old are also at risk.

Race can also play a role in COVID-19 risk. The **CDC** found that 33 percent of Americans hospitalized with COVID-19 were African American. However, only 13 percent of the US population is African American.

Experts believe there are many possible reasons for this imbalance. One is that African Americans are more likely to have existing

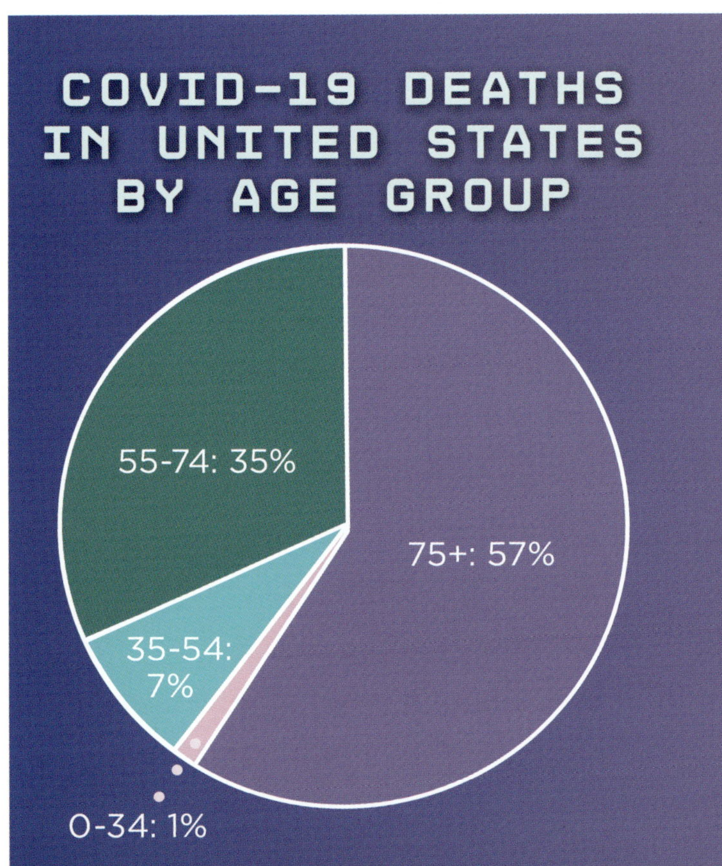

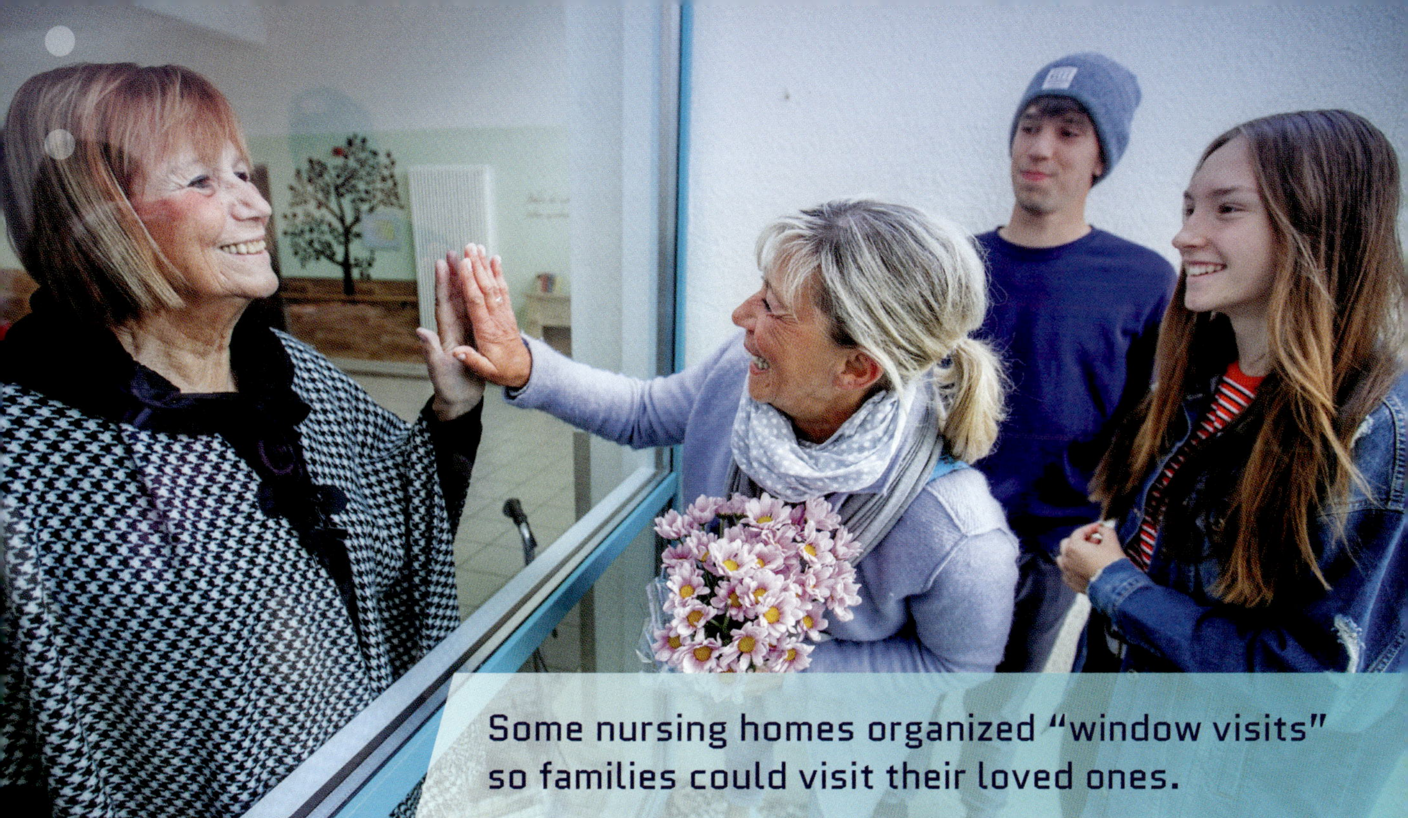
Some nursing homes organized "window visits" so families could visit their loved ones.

health conditions. African Americans are also more likely to face **discrimination** and other **barriers** that make it difficult to get high-paying jobs. In low-paying jobs, social distancing is often difficult. So, African Americans are more likely to be exposed to the coronavirus.

Most people who caught COVID-19 recovered. However, the number of **infections** and deaths was high. By early June, there were nearly 6.4 million confirmed cases worldwide. Of these, more than 380,000 were fatal.

Health Crisis

US hospitals were soon overwhelmed with COVID-19 patients. Many hospitals canceled all nonemergency medical procedures. This allowed doctors and nurses to spend more time treating COVID-19 patients.

Another solution was to set up temporary hospitals in other buildings. New York City had one of the highest rates of COVID-19 in the United States. In April, a 350-bed hospital was set up inside the Billie Jean King National Tennis Center in Queens.

But, staffing hospitals was a problem. Doctors and nurses had to work long hours. Many healthcare workers fell ill with COVID-19 and couldn't work. New York and other hard-hit states asked retired doctors to help. But staff and space **shortages** weren't the only **barriers** to treating COVID-19 patients.

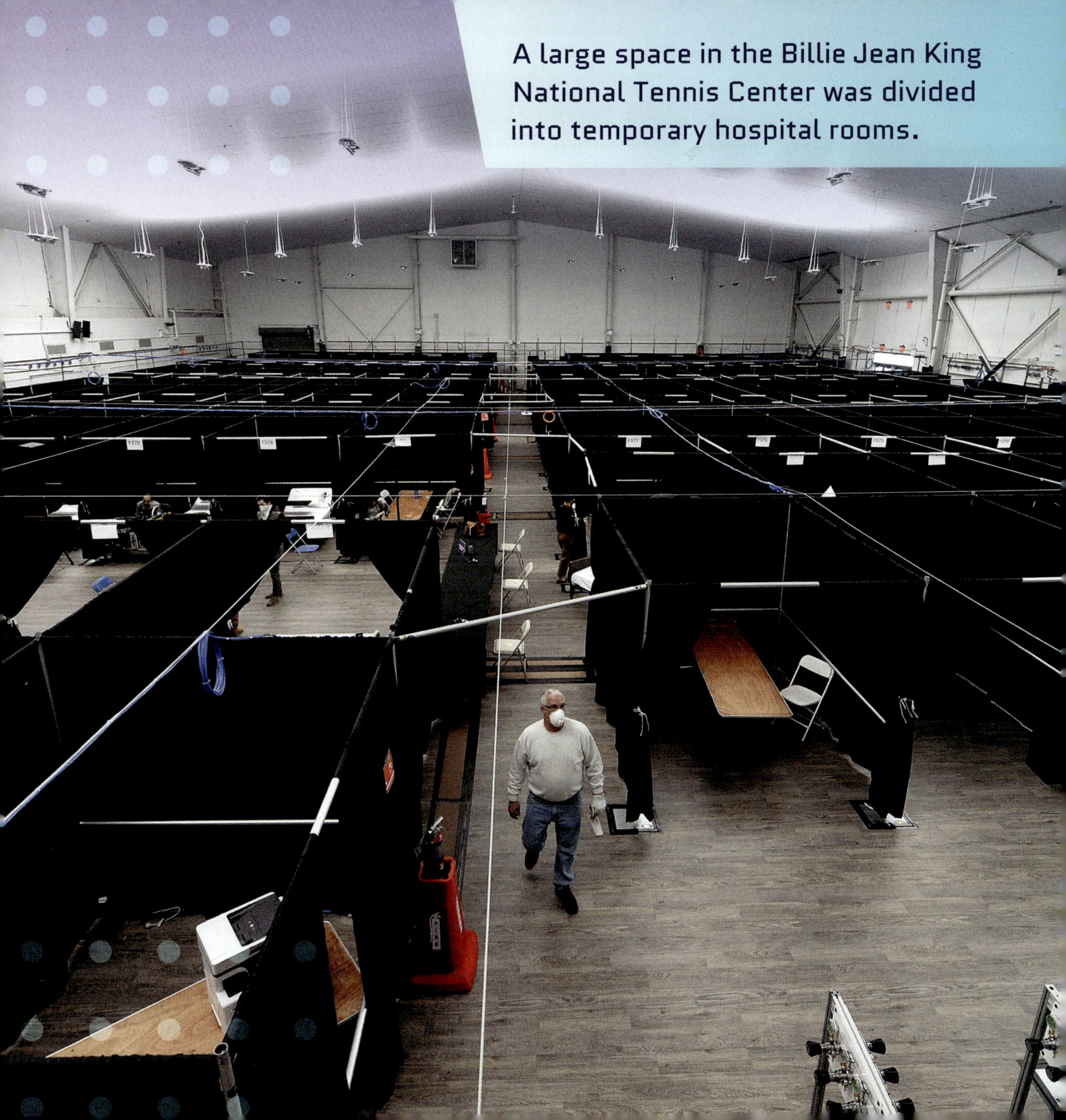

A large space in the Billie Jean King National Tennis Center was divided into temporary hospital rooms.

Supply Shortages

The United States and many other countries were not prepared for the COVID-19 **crisis.** These countries did not have enough personal protective equipment (PPE) available. PPE includes face masks, gloves, and gowns. Healthcare workers need PPE to protect themselves and their patients from **infections**.

US hospitals often bought PPE from China. But during the **pandemic**, China needed more PPE for its own healthcare workers. Chinese factories also made less PPE as employees became sick and couldn't work. So, less PPE was sold to the United States.

Ventilators were also in short supply. These machines push oxygen into patients' lungs. This helps the patients breathe. Difficulty breathing is a main **symptom** of COVID-19. So, many more ventilators were suddenly needed.

STEM CONNECTION

Some hospitals were able to use modified BiPAP devices to treat less-critical COVID-19 patients. These simple breathing machines use pressurized air to keep people's airways open.

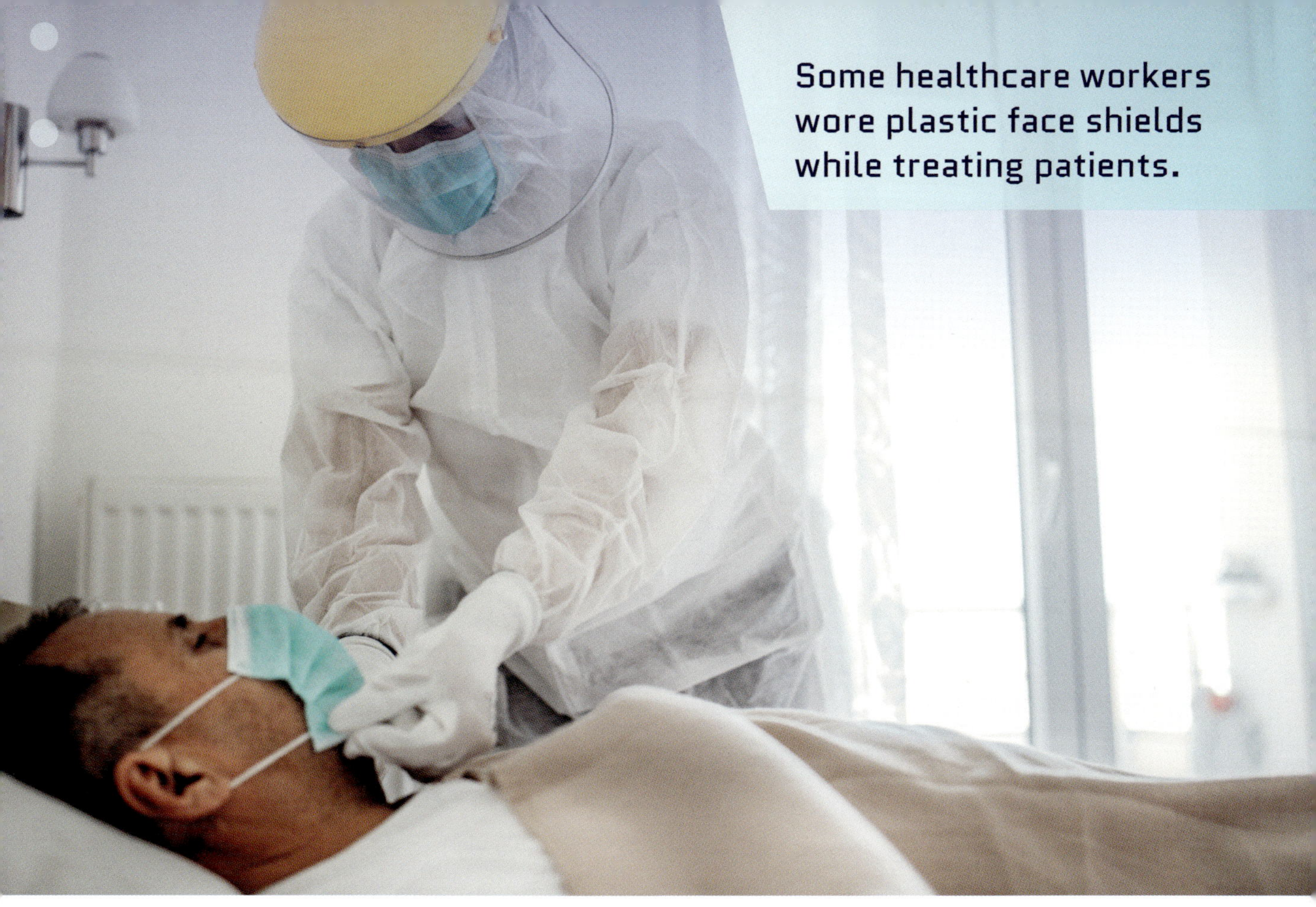

Some healthcare workers wore plastic face shields while treating patients.

Many different US companies worked to make PPE and ventilators in their factories. Despite these efforts, most hospitals still didn't have enough PPE. And, healthcare workers weren't the only people who needed it. Many workers at **essential** businesses also didn't have face masks or gloves. So, they were at greater risk of catching COVID-19. The lack of PPE added stress and confusion to the **pandemic**.

Staying Informed

Staying informed about the pandemic was also stressful and confusing for many people. Leaders across the United States did their best to keep people informed. However, the situation changed from day to day. This made it difficult for people to know what information was correct.

For example, different news outlets provided conflicting information about the pandemic. So, Americans disagreed about the pandemic's severity. As a result, some people protested stay-at-home orders. They felt that the **restrictions** were too high a price to pay to control the spread of COVID-19.

Also, responses to the spread of COVID-19 varied from state to state. Some governors imposed stay-at-home restrictions sooner than others. And, some states lifted their orders sooner than others. This led to confusion and arguments over the right action to take.

However, many people wanted to continue social distancing until COVID-19 was under control. This was supported by the **WHO**, the **CDC**, and most other healthcare officials.

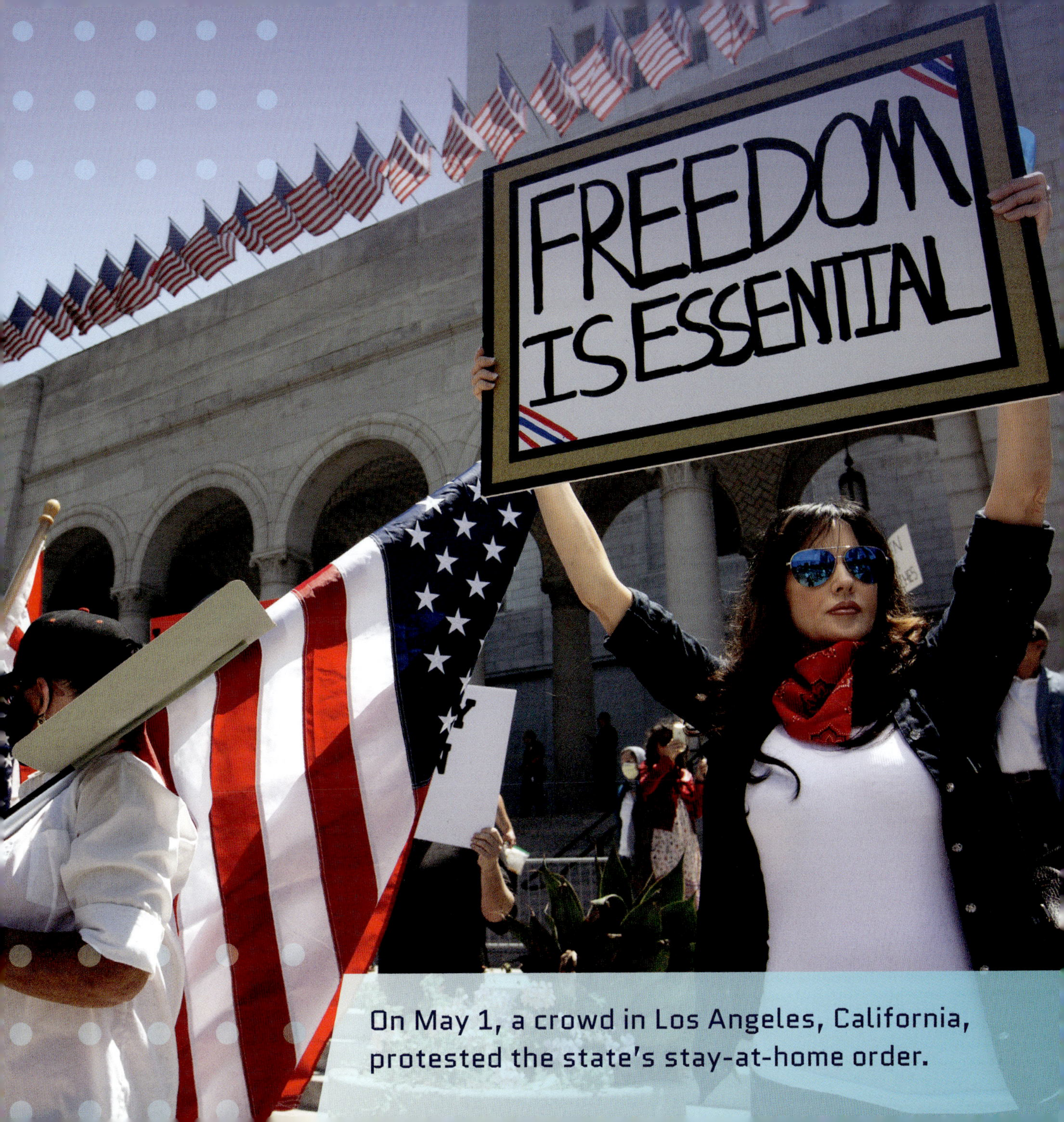

On May 1, a crowd in Los Angeles, California, protested the state's stay-at-home order.

Looking Toward the Future

No one knew how long the COVID-19 **pandemic** would last. So, US citizens and leaders had to figure out short-term answers. Over the summer, many states allowed businesses to reopen. However, this led to a sharp increase in COVID-19 cases in some places. So, many businesses had to close again.

By October 2020, the virus had **infected** 33 million people. One million had died. The world hoped scientists could create a COVID-19 vaccine. This would prevent people from getting the disease.

Hundreds of medical companies were testing COVID-19 vaccines. But the vaccine testing process takes a long time. Scientists have to make sure a vaccine will work without causing other problems. By December 2020, several vaccines were nearing approval. Experts believed at least two vaccines would be available in the United States by the end of the year.

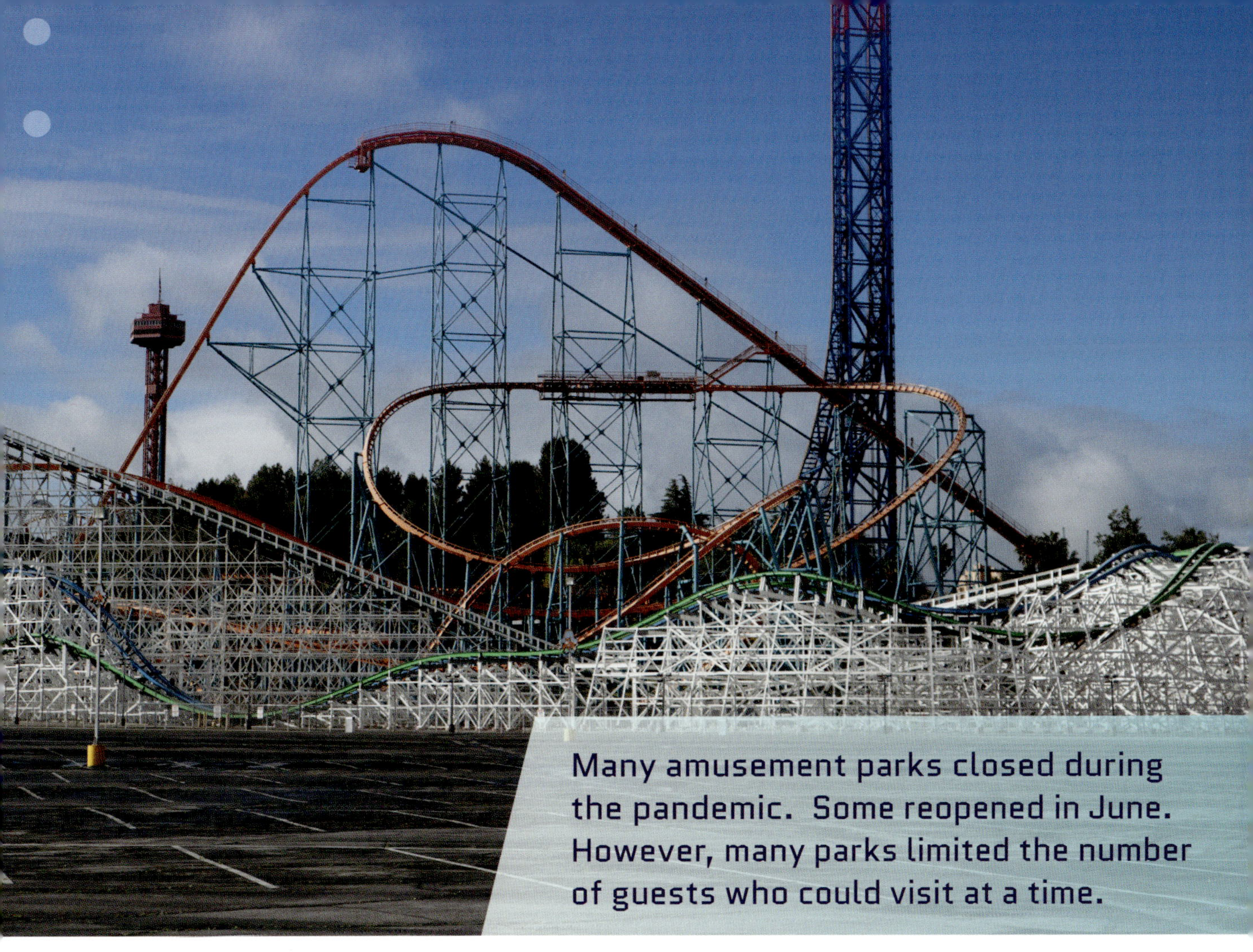

Many amusement parks closed during the pandemic. Some reopened in June. However, many parks limited the number of guests who could visit at a time.

In the meantime, Americans were encouraged to wear face masks and maintain social distance when in public. This was the best way for people to keep themselves and others safe as the **pandemic** continued.

Glossary

antibody—a substance produced by special cells of the body to fight an attack, such as by a disease or an allergen.

asthma—a condition that causes wheezing and coughing and makes breathing difficult.

barrier—anything that makes progress difficult.

Centers for Disease Control and Prevention (CDC)—the main national health organization in the United States. The CDC works to control the spread of disease and maintain and improve public health in the United States and other countries.

crisis—a difficult or dangerous situation that needs serious attention.

discrimination (dihs-krih-muh-NAY-shuhn)—unfair treatment, often based on race, religion, or gender.

essential—very important or necessary.

infection—an unhealthy condition caused by something harmful, such as a virus. If something has an infection, it is infected.

lockdown—a temporary measure ordered by government officials in which people are required to stay at home and limit public contact.

originate—to create or begin.

outbreak—a sudden increase in the occurrence of an illness.

pandemic—worldwide spread of a disease that can affect most people.

respiratory—having to do with the system of organs involved with breathing.

restrict—to keep within certain limits. Something that does this is a restriction.

shortage—a lack of something that is needed.

symptom—a noticeable change in the normal working of the body. A symptom indicates or accompanies disease, sickness, or another malfunction.

World Health Organization (WHO)—an agency of the United Nations that works to maintain and improve the health of people around the world.

Online Resources

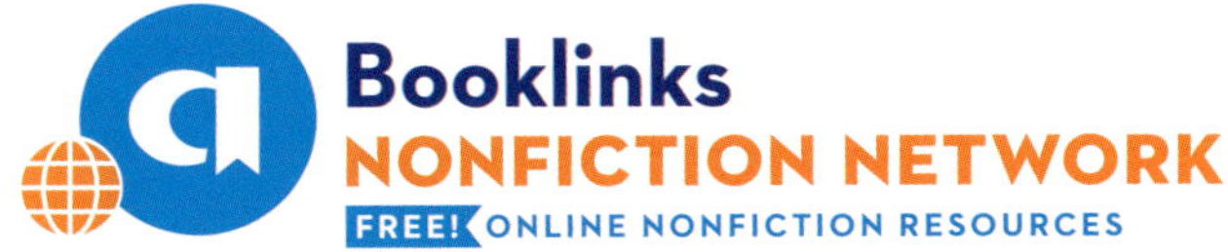

To learn more about the COVID-19 pandemic, please visit **abdobooklinks.com** or scan this QR code. These links are routinely monitored and updated to provide the most current information available.

Index